ALCOHOLICS
ANONYMOUS

ALCOHOLICS ANONYMOUS

The Landmark of
Recovery and Vital Living

Newly Abridged and Introduced by
Mitch Horowitz

THE CONDENSED CLASSICS LIBRARY™

Published by Gildan Media LLC
aka G&D Media.
www.GandDmedia.com

Alcoholics Anonymous was originally published in 1939
G&D Media Condensed Classics edition published 2018
Abridgement and Introduction copyright © 2016 by Mitch
Horowitz

No part of this book may be reproduced or transmitted in any
form, by any means, (electronic, photocopying, recording, or
otherwise) without the prior written permission of the author.
No liability is assumed with respect to the use of the information
contained within. Although every precaution has been taken, the
author and publisher assume no liability for errors or omissions.
Neither is any liability assumed for damages resulting from the
use of the information contained herein.

FIRST EDITION: 2018

Cover design by David Rheinhardt of Pyrographx

Interior design by Meghan Day Healey of Story Horse, LLC.

ISBN: 978-1-7225-0048-1

CONTENTS

Abridging a Sacred Text

You are about to encounter an abridgment of probably the greatest work of modern self-help. That *Alcoholics Anonymous* has saved and revitalized countless lives since its initial publication in 1939 does not require excessive restatement here. More important is that some readers who have experienced the power of this book would understandably chaff at the notion of its abridgement. To some, *Alcoholics Anonymous* is a work of almost Scriptural significance, and condensing it can seem like an act of heresy, if not cynicism.

I can promise you that my motive is neither. As a writer, historian, and seeker, I approach this book on bended knee, and with deepest gratitude. I consider it the most effective program of spiritual self-help of the past hundred years, and perhaps beyond. My intent in condensing this work is not to replace or sidestep the complete version of the "Big Book," which I encourage you to read. My aim, rather, is to supply a resource for people who may be unready to dive into the Big Book but can be induced by this shorter and equally faithful journey. This condensed edition is also for veterans of the Big Book who wish to review or reencounter its core points. Whatever brings you to this edition, you can experience its ideas in about an hour of reading or listening. Is the length of a lunch break, or a morning commute, too much to dedicate to a philosophy of self-development that can change everything for you, or for someone you love?

Alcoholics Anonymous was written for alcoholics and their loved ones—but it is not for them alone. As readers and self-improvers have repeatedly discovered, the "twelve steps" of *Alcoholics Anonymous*, which are described in chapter four, are a blueprint that can be applied to virtually life-depleting habit or compulsion, such as anger, gambling, drugs, debt-spending, or chronic overeating. Although the book was written by and for those who struggle with alcohol, nearly any term or problem, like the ones I just named, can be substituted wherever the word alcohol appears.

What is an addiction? The brilliant actor Philip Seymour Hoffman, who died of a drug overdose in 2014, told a friend that "addiction is when you do the

thing you really, really most don't want to be doing."
Whatever repeatedly derails your life, threatens your
health, and distracts you from your finest and highest tasks, represents an addiction or compulsion. The
twelve-step program can direct you to fuller (and safer)
existence, whatever the problem that keeps you from it.

As I consider the responsibility of abridging a work
that has saved lives, reassembled broken households,
and redirected people from paths leading to illness and
despair, I am reminded of a recent exchange I had with
a successful self-help writer. He told me that he didn't
regard himself as a self-help writer at all. He considered the label gauche, and called most self-help books
a sham.

In my twenty years as a writer, publisher, and user
of self-help philosophies, I have heard that attitude
often. It comes not infrequently from self-help writers
themselves, some of whom aspire to traditional conceptions of literary recognition, and fear that the label
detracts from their respectability or seriousness. I have
also, and more often, heard such judgments from people who are looking for reasons to avoid books like this
one, suspecting that its program will remake them into
ineffectual, woo-woo automatons, unsuited to the rig-
ors of commerce, artistry, or professionalism. Nothing
could be further from the truth.

This book provides a restoration of the path toward life—and away from pettiness, compulsion, and self-destruction. Its path is, unashamedly, one of power. Not the kind of ersatz power that we seek from our self-will. If will power worked, there would be no addicts or alcoholics. Rather, this book directs you toward the power derived from having a relationship with the Highest Source of life. Do you reject or have difficulty conceiving of a Higher Power? That is no barrier to entry. The authors of *Alcoholics Anonymous* dealt with the question of belief in an intellectually serious and non-dogmatic way. They placed no ideological tollgate in front of anyone seeking help. They asked only for sincerity of intent.

In any case, my point is not to sell you on the effectiveness of this or any self-help program. Only you can make that evaluation. Rather, I wish to encourage you, as you begin this book, to understand that labels are secondary and ideas alone matter. The only measure of a practical philosophy is its efficacy. A high-sounding ethical or spiritual idea that doesn't work for the individual is worse than useless.

One word of caution: The methods and principles in this book reveal themselves only to someone who approaches them with deep seriousness. The requirements of the twelve-steps are simple but not cheap. They call for a special kind of dedication, a willingness to work with others, and a policy of zero-tolerance for cynicism, eye-rolling, or self-justification. If you can bring that kind of the commitment to the table, the twelve-steps will serve you as a life-changing resource. Of that much I am certain.

—Mitch Horowitz

The Doctor's Opinion

Men and women drink essentially because they like the effect produced by alcohol. To them, their alcoholic life seems the only normal one. They are restless, irritable, and discontented, unless they can again experience the sense of ease and comfort that comes at once by taking a few drinks—drinks which they see others taking with impunity. After they have succumbed to the desire again, as so many do, and the phenomenon of craving develops, they pass through the well-known stages of a spree, emerging remorseful, with a firm resolution not to drink again. This is repeated over and over, and unless this person can experience an entire psychic change there is very little hope of his recovery.

On the other hand—and strange as this may seem to those who do not understand—once a psychic change has occurred, the very same person who seemed doomed, who had so many problems he despaired of ever solving them, suddenly finds himself easily able to control his desire for alcohol, the only effort necessary being that required to follow a few simple rules.

Men have cried out to me in sincere and despairing appeal: "Doctor, I cannot go on like this! I have everything to live for! I must stop, but I cannot! You must help me!"

Faced with this problem, if a doctor is honest with himself, he must sometimes feel his own inadequacy. Although he gives all that is in him, it often is not enough. One feels that something more than human power is needed to produce the essential psychic change. Though the aggregate of recoveries resulting from psychiatric effort is considerable, we physicians must admit we have made little impression upon the problem as a whole. Many types do not respond to the ordinary psychological approach.

I do not hold with those who believe that alcoholism is entirely a problem of mental control. I have had many men who had, for example, worked a period of months on some problem or business deal, which was to be settled on a certain date, favorably to them. They took a drink a day or so prior to the date, and then the phenomenon of craving at once became paramount to all other interests so that the important appointment was not met. These men were not drinking to escape; they were drinking to overcome a craving beyond their mental control.

There is the type of man who is unwilling to admit that he cannot take a drink. He plans various ways of drinking. He changes his brand or his environment. There is the type who always believes that after being entirely free from alcohol for a period of time he can take a drink without danger. There is the manic-depressive type, who is, perhaps, the least understood by his friends, and about whom a whole chapter could be written. Then there are types entirely normal in every respect except in the effect alcohol has upon them. They are often able, intelligent, friendly people.

All these, and many others, have one symptom in common: they cannot start drinking without developing the phenomenon of craving. This phenomenon has never been, by any treatment with which we are familiar, permanently eradicated. The only relief we have to suggest is entire abstinence.

When I need a mental uplift, I often think of a case brought in by a physician prominent in New York City. The patient had made his own diagnosis, and deciding his situation hopeless, had hidden in a deserted barn determined to die. He was rescued by a searching party, and, in desperate condition, brought to me. Following his physical rehabilitation, he had a talk with me in which he frankly stated he thought the treatment a waste of effort, unless I could assure him, which no one ever had, that in the future he would have the "will power" to resist the impulse to drink.

His alcoholic problem was so complex, and his depression so great, that we felt his only hope would be through what we then called "moral psychology," and we doubted if even that would have any effect. However, he did become "sold" on the ideas contained in this book. He has not had a drink for more than three years.

I earnestly advise every alcoholic to read this book through, and though perhaps he came to scoff, he may remain to pray.

CHAPTER ONE

Bill's Story

War fever ran high in the New England town to which we new, young officers were assigned, and we were flattered when the first citizens took us to their homes, making us feel heroic. I forgot the strong warnings and the prejudices of my people concerning drink. In time we sailed for "Over There." I was very lonely and again turned to alcohol.

At twenty-two, and a veteran of foreign wars, I returned home at last. My talent for leadership, I imagined, would place me at the head of vast enterprises, which I would manage with utmost assurance.

I took a night law course, and obtained employment as investigator for a surety company. The drive for success was on. I'd prove to the world I was important. My work took me about Wall Street and little by little I became interested in the market. Many people lost money—but some became very rich. Why not I? I stud-

ied economics and business as well as law. Potential alcoholic that I was, I nearly failed my law course. At one
of the finals I was too drunk to think or write. Though
my drinking was not yet continuous, it disturbed my
wife.

By the time I had completed the course, I knew the
law was not for me. Wall Street had me in its grip. Business and financial leaders were my heroes. I failed to
persuade my broker friends to send me out looking over
factories and managements, but my wife and I decided
to go anyway. I had developed a theory that most people lost money in stocks through ignorance of markets.
I discovered many more reasons later on.

We gave up our positions and off we roared on a
motorcycle, the sidecar stuffed with tent, blankets,
change of clothes, and three huge volumes of a financial
reference service.

For the next few years fortune threw money and
applause my way. My judgment and ideas were followed
by many to the tune of paper millions.

Meanwhile, my drinking assumed more serious
proportions, continuing all day and almost every night.
The remonstrances of my friends terminated in a row
and I became a lone wolf. There were many unhappy
scenes in our apartment.

I began to be jittery in the morning.

Abruptly in October 1929 hell broke loose on the New York stock exchange. After one of those days of inferno, I was finished and so were many friends. The papers reported men jumping to death from the towers of High Finance. That disgusted me. I would not jump. I went back to the bar. My friends had dropped several million—so what? As I drank, the old fierce determination to win came back.

Our resources drained, we went to live with my wife's parents. I found a job; then lost it as the result of a brawl with a taxi driver. Mercifully, no one could guess that I was to have no real employment for five years, or hardly draw a sober breath. My wife began to work in a department store, coming home exhausted to find me drunk. I became an unwelcome hanger-on at brokerage places. Liquor became a necessity.

Sometimes a small deal would net a few hundred dollars, and I would pay my bills at the bars and delicatessens. This went on endlessly, and I began to waken very early in the morning shaking violently. A tumbler full of gin followed by half a dozen bottles of beer would be required if I were to eat any breakfast. Nevertheless, I still thought I could control the situation, and there were periods of sobriety which renewed my wife's hope.

Gradually things got worse. The house was taken over by the mortgage holder, my mother-in-law died, my wife and father-in-law became ill. Then I got a promising business opportunity. Stocks were at the low point of 1932, and I had somehow formed a group to buy. I was to share generously in the profits. I went on a prodigious bender, and that chance vanished.

This had to stop. I saw I could not take so much as one drink. I was through forever. Before then, I had written lots of sweet promises, but my wife happily observed that this time I meant business. And so I did. Shortly afterward I came home drunk. There had been no fight. Where had been my high resolve? I simply didn't know. It hadn't even come to mind. Someone had pushed a drink my way, and I had taken it. Was I crazy? I began to wonder, for such an appalling lack of perspective seemed near being just that.

Renewing my resolve, I tried again. Some time passed, and confidence began to be replaced by cocksureness. I could laugh at the gin mills. Now I had what it takes! One day I walked into a cafe to use the telephone. In no time I was beating on the bar asking myself how it happened. As the whiskey rose to my head I told myself I would manage better *next time*.

The remorse, horror, and hopelessness of the next morning are unforgettable. The courage to do battle was not there. My brain raced uncontrollably and there was a terrible sense of impending calamity. Should I kill myself? No—not now. Then a mental fog settled down. Gin would fix that. So two bottles, and—oblivion.

The mind and body are marvelous mechanisms, for mine endured this agony two more years. Sometimes I stole from my wife's slender purse when the morning terror and madness were on me. Again I swayed dizzily before an open window, or the medicine cabinet where there was poison, cursing myself for a weakling. Then came the night when the physical and mental torture was so hellish I feared I would burst through my window. Somehow I managed to drag my mattress to a lower floor, lest I suddenly leap. Next day found me drinking both gin and sedative.

I could eat little or nothing when drinking, and I was forty pounds underweight.

My brother-in-law is a physician, and through his kindness and that of my mother I was placed in a nationally known hospital for the mental and physical rehabilitation of alcoholics. Under the so-called belladonna treatment my brain cleared. Hydrotherapy and mild exercise helped.

The frightful day came when I drank once more. After a time I returned to the hospital. This was the finish, the curtain, it seemed to me. My weary and despairing wife was informed that she would soon have to give me over to the undertaker or the asylum.

No words can tell of the loneliness and despair I found in that bitter morass of self-pity. Quicksand stretched around me in all directions. I had met my match. Alcohol was my master. Trembling, I stepped from the hospital a broken man. Fear sobered me for a bit. Then came the insidious insanity of that first drink, and on Armistice Day 1934, I was off again. Everyone became resigned to the certainty that I would have to be shut up somewhere, or would stumble along to a miserable end.

How dark it is before the dawn! In reality that was the beginning of my last debauch. I was soon catapulted into what I like to call the fourth dimension of existence. I was to know happiness, peace, and usefulness, in a way of life that is incredibly more wonderful as time passes.

Near the end of that bleak November, I sat drinking in my kitchen. With a certain satisfaction I reflected there was enough gin concealed about the house to carry me through that night and the next day. My musing was interrupted by the telephone. The cheery voice of an old school friend asked if he might come over. *He was sober.* It was years since I could remember his coming to New York in that condition. I was amazed. Rumor had it that he had been committed for alcoholic insanity. I wondered how he had escaped. Of course he would have dinner, and then I could drink openly with him. Unmindful of his welfare, I thought only of recapturing the spirit of other days.

The door opened and he stood there, fresh-skinned and glowing. There was something about his eyes. He was inexplicably different. What had happened? I pushed a drink across the table. He refused it. Disappointed but curious, I wondered what had got into him. "What's all this about?" I queried. He looked straight at me. Simply, but smilingly, he said, "I've got religion."

I was aghast. So that was it—last summer an alcoholic crackpot; now, I suspected, a little cracked about religion. He had that starry-eyed look. Yes, the old boy was on fire all right. But bless his heart, let him rant! Besides, my gin would last longer than his preaching. But he did no ranting. In a matter of fact way he told how two men had appeared in court, persuading the judge to suspend his commitment. They had told of a simple religious idea and a practical program of action. That was two months ago and the result was self evident. It worked!

He had come to pass his experience along to me— if I cared to have it. I was shocked, but interested. I had always believed in a power greater than myself. I had often pondered these things. I was not an atheist. My intellectual heroes, the chemists, the astronomers, even the evolutionists, suggested vast laws and forces at work. Despite contrary indications, I had little doubt that a mighty purpose and rhythm underlay all. How could there be so much of precise and immutable law, and no intelligence? I simply had to believe in a Spirit of the Universe, who knew neither time nor limitation. But that was as far as I had gone.

With ministers, and the world's religions, I parted right there. When they talked of a God personal to me, who was love, superhuman strength, and direction, I became irritated and my mind snapped shut against such a theory. To Christ I conceded the certainty of a great man. His moral teaching—most excellent. For myself, I had adopted those parts that seemed convenient and not too difficult; the rest I disregarded. The wars, the burnings, and chicanery that religious dispute had facilitated made me sick. I doubted whether, on balance, the religions of mankind had done any good. Judging from what I had seen in Europe and since, the power of God in human affairs was negligible, the Brotherhood of Man a grim jest.

But my friend sat before me, and he made the point-blank declaration that God had done for him what he could not do for himself. That he had, in effect, been raised from the dead, suddenly taken from the scrap heap to a level of life better than the best he had ever known! Had this power originated in him? Obviously it had not. There had been no more power in him than there was in me at that minute; and this was none at all.

That floored me. It began to look as though religious people were right after all. Here was something at work in a human heart that had done the impossible. My ideas about miracles were drastically revised right then. Never mind the musty past; here sat a miracle directly across the kitchen table.

I saw that my friend was much more than inwardly reorganized. He was on a different footing. Despite the living example of my friend there remained in me vestiges of my old prejudice. The word God still aroused a certain antipathy. When the thought was expressed that there might be a God personal to me this feeling was intensified. I didn't like the idea. I could go for such conceptions as Creative Intelligence, Universal Mind or Spirit of Nature, but I resisted the thought of a Czar of the Heavens however loving His sway might be. I have since talked with scores of men who felt the same.

My friend suggested what then seemed a novel idea. He said, *"Why don't you choose your own conception of God?"* That statement hit me hard.

It was only a matter of being willing to believe in a power greater than myself. Nothing more was required of me to make my beginning. I saw that growth could start from that point.

Thus was I convinced that God is concerned with us humans when we want Him enough. At long last I saw, I felt, I believed. Scales of pride and prejudice fell from my eyes. A new world came into view.

At the hospital I was separated from alcohol for the last time. Treatment seemed wise, for I showed signs of delirium tremens. There I humbly offered myself to God, as I then understood Him, to do with me as He would. I placed myself unreservedly under His care and direction. I admitted for the first time that of myself I was nothing. I ruthlessly faced my sins and became willing to have my newfound Friend take them away, root and branch. I have not had a drink since.

My schoolmate visited me, and I fully acquainted him with my problems and deficiencies. We made a list of people I had hurt or toward whom I felt resentment. I expressed my entire willingness to approach these individuals, admitting my wrong. Never was I to be critical of them. I was to right all such matters to the utmost of my ability.

I was to test my thinking by the new God-consciousness within. Common sense would thus become uncommon sense. I was to sit quietly when in doubt, asking only for direction and strength to meet my problems as He would have me. Never was I to pray for myself, except as my requests bore on my usefulness to others. Then only might I expect to receive. But that would be in great measure.

My friend promised when these things were done I would enter upon a new relationship with my Creator; that I would have the elements of a way of living, which answered all my problems. Belief in the power of God, plus enough willingness, honesty and humility to establish and maintain the new order of things, were the essential requirements.

Simple, but not easy; a price had to be paid. It meant destruction of self-centeredness. I must turn in all things to the Father of Lights who presides over us all.

These were revolutionary and drastic proposals, but the moment I fully accepted them, the effect was electric. There was a sense of victory, followed by such a peace and serenity as I had never known. There was utter confidence. I felt lifted up, as though the great clean wind of a mountaintop blew through and through. God comes to most men gradually, but His impact on me was sudden and profound.

Alarmed for my sanity, I called my friend the doctor. He listened in wonder as I talked. Finally he shook his head saying, "Something has happened to you that I don't understand. But you had better hang on to it.

Anything is better than the way you were." The good doctor now sees many men who have such experiences. He knows they are real.

While I lay in the hospital, the thought came that there were thousands of hopeless alcoholics who might be glad to have what had been so freely given me. Perhaps I could help some of them. They, in turn, might work with others. My friend had emphasized the absolute necessity of demonstrating these principles in all my affairs. It was particularly imperative to work with others as he had worked with me. Faith without works was dead, he said. And how appallingly true for the alcoholic! For if an alcoholic failed to perfect and enlarge his spiritual life through work and self sacrifice for others, he could not survive the certain trials and low spots ahead.

My wife and I abandoned ourselves with enthusiasm to the idea of helping other alcoholics to a solution of their problems. We commenced to make many fast friends and a fellowship has grown up among us. Most of us feel we need look no further for Utopia. We have it with us right here and now. Each day my friend's simple talk in our kitchen multiplies itself in a widening circle of peace on earth and good will.

CHAPTER TWO

There Is a Solution

We of Alcoholics Anonymous know countless people who were once just as hopeless as Bill. All have recovered. They have solved the drink problem.

We are average Americans. We are people who normally would not mix. But there exists among us a fellowship, a friendliness, and an understanding, which is indescribably wonderful. We are like the passengers of a great liner the moment after rescue from shipwreck when camaraderie, joyousness and democracy pervade the vessel from steerage to captain's table. Unlike the feelings of the ship's passengers, however, our joy in escape from disaster does not subside as we go our individual ways. The feeling of having shared in a common peril is one element in the powerful cement that binds us. But that in itself would never have held us together as we are now joined.

The tremendous fact for every one of us is that we have discovered a common solution. This is the great news this book carries to those who suffer from alcoholism.

An illness of this sort—and we have come to believe it an illness—involves those about us in a way no other human sickness can. If a person has cancer all are sorry for him and no one is angry or hurt. But not so with the alcoholic illness, for with it there goes annihilation of all the things worthwhile in life. It engulfs all whose lives touch the sufferer's. We hope this volume will inform and comfort those who are, or who may be affected.

Highly competent psychiatrists who have dealt with us found it sometimes impossible to persuade an alcoholic to discuss his situation without reserve. *But the ex-alcoholic who has found this solution, who is properly armed with facts about himself, can generally win the entire confidence of another alcoholic in a few hours. Until such an understanding is reached, little or nothing can be accomplished.*

How many times people have said to us: "I can take it or leave it. Why can't he?" "Why don't you try beer and wine?" "Lay off the hard stuff." "His will power must be weak." "He could stop if he wanted to." "The doctor told him that if he ever drank again it would kill him, but there he is lit up again."

These are commonplace observations on drinkers which we hear all the time. Back of them is a world of ignorance and misunderstanding. We see that these expressions refer to people whose reactions are very different from ours.

Moderate drinkers have little trouble in giving up liquor entirely if they have good reason for it. They can take it or leave it alone. Then we have a certain type of hard drinker. He may have the habit badly enough to gradually impair himself physically and mentally. It may cause him to die a few years before his time. If a sufficiently strong reason—ill health, falling in love, change of environment, or the warning of a doctor— becomes operative, this man can also stop or moderate, although he may find it difficult and troublesome, and may even need medical attention.

But what about the real alcoholic? He may start off as a moderate drinker; he may or may not become a continuous hard drinker; but at some stage of his drinking career he begins to lose all control of his liquor consumption once he starts to drink.

He may be one of the finest fellows in the world. Yet let him drink for a day, and he frequently becomes disgustingly, and even dangerously, anti-social. He has a positive genius for getting tight at exactly the wrong moment, particularly when some important decision must be made or engagement kept. He is often perfectly sensible and well balanced concerning everything except liquor, but in that respect is incredibly dishonest and selfish.

Why does he behave like this? If hundreds of experiences have shown him that one drink means another debacle with all its attendant suffering and humiliation, why is it he takes that one drink? What has become of the common sense and will power that he still sometimes displays with respect to other matters?

Opinions vary considerably as to why the alcoholic reacts differently from normal people. We are not sure why, once a certain point is reached, little can be done for him. We cannot answer the riddle.

We know that while the alcoholic keeps away from drink, as he may do for months or years, he reacts much like other men. We are equally positive that once he takes any alcohol whatever into his system, something happens, both in the bodily and mental sense, which makes it virtually impossible for him to stop.

The fact is that most alcoholics, for reasons yet obscure, have lost the power of choice in drink. Our so-called will power becomes practically non-existent. We are unable at certain times, to bring into our consciousness with sufficient force the memory of the suffering and humiliation of even a week or a month ago. We are without defense against the first drink.

There *is* a solution. Almost none of us liked the self-searching, the leveling of our pride, the confession of shortcomings, which the process requires for its successful consummation. But we saw that it really worked in others, and we had come to believe in the hopelessness and futility of life as we had been living it. When, therefore, we were approached by those in whom the problem had been solved, there was nothing left for us but to pick up the simple kit of spiritual tools laid at our feet. We have found much of heaven and we have been rocketed into a fourth dimension of existence, of which we had not even dreamed.

The great fact is just this, and nothing less: that we have had deep and effective spiritual experiences, which have revolutionized our whole attitude toward life, toward our fellows, and toward God's universe. The central fact of our lives today is the absolute certainty that our Creator has entered into our hearts and lives in a way that is indeed miraculous. He has commenced to accomplish those things for us that we could never do by ourselves.

If you are as seriously alcoholic as we were, we believe there is no middle-of-the-road solution. We were in a position where life was becoming impossible, and if we had passed into the region from which there is no return through human aid, we had but two alternatives: one was to go on to the bitter end, blotting out the consciousness of our intolerable situation as best we could; and the other, to accept spiritual help. This we did because we honestly wanted to, and were willing to make the effort.

A certain American businessman had ability, good sense, and high character. For years he had floundered from one sanitarium to another. He had consulted the best known American psychiatrists. Then he had gone to Europe, placing himself in the care of a celebrated physician who prescribed for him.

He wished above all things to regain self-control. He seemed quite rational and well-balanced with respect to other problems. Yet he had no control whatever over alcohol. Why was this?

He begged the doctor to tell him the whole truth, and he got it. In the doctor's judgment he was utterly hopeless; he could never regain his position in society and he would have to place himself under lock and key, or hire a bodyguard if he expected to live long.

But this man still lives, and is a free man. He does not need a bodyguard, nor is he confined. He can go anywhere on earth without disaster, provided he remains willing to maintain a certain simple attitude. Let us tell you the rest of the conversation our friend had with his doctor.

The doctor said: "You have the mind of a chronic alcoholic. I have never seen one single case recover, where that state of mind existed to the extent that it does in you." Our friend felt as though the gates of hell had closed on him.

He said to the doctor, "Is there no exception?"

"Yes," replied the doctor, "there is. Exceptions to cases such as yours have been occurring since early times. Here and there, once in a while, alcoholics have had what are called vital spiritual experiences. To me these occurrences are phenomena. They appear to be in the nature of huge emotional displacements and re-arrangements. Ideas, emotions, and attitudes, which were once the guiding forces of the lives of these men, are suddenly cast to one side, and a completely new set of conceptions and motives begin to dominate them. In fact, I have been trying to produce some such emotional rearrangement within you. With many individuals the methods which I employed are successful, but I have never been successful with an alcoholic of your description."

Upon hearing this our friend was somewhat relieved, for he reflected that, after all, he was a good church member. This hope, however, was destroyed by the doctor's telling him that his religious convictions were very good, but that in his case they did not spell the necessary vital spiritual experience.

Here was the terrible dilemma in which our friend found himself when he had the extraordinary experience, which as we have already told you, made him a free man.

We, in our turn, sought the same escape, with all the desperation of drowning men. What seemed at first a flimsy reed, has proved to be the loving and powerful hand of God. A new life has been given us or, if you prefer, "a design for living" that really works.

The distinguished American psychologist, William James, in his book *Varieties of Religious Experience* indicates a multitude of ways in which men have discovered God. We have no desire to convince anyone that there is only one way by which faith can be acquired. If what we have learned, and felt, and seen, means anything at all, it means that all of us are the children of a living Creator with whom we may form a relationship upon simple and understandable terms as soon as we are willing and honest enough to try. Those having religious affiliations will find here nothing disturbing to their beliefs or ceremonies. There is no friction among us over such matters.

*   *   *

One more word about the outlook of the alcoholic. The idea that somehow, someday he will control and enjoy his liquor drinking is the great obsession of every abnormal drinker. It may be true that certain non-alcoholic people, though drinking foolishly and heavily at the present time, are able to stop or moderate. But the actual or potential alcoholic, with hardly an exception, will be *absolutely unable to stop drinking on the basis of self-knowledge.*

Many doctors and psychiatrists agree with our conclusions. One of them, a staff member of a world-renowned hospital, recently made this statement to some of us: "What you say about the general hopelessness of the average alcoholic's plight is, in my opinion, correct. As to two of you men, whose stories I have heard, there is no doubt in my mind that you were 100% hopeless, apart from Divine help. Had you offered yourselves as patients at this hospital, I would not have taken you, if I had been able to avoid it. People like you are too heartbreaking. Though not a religious person, I have profound respect for the spiritual approach in such cases as yours. For most cases, there is virtually no other solution."

Once more: the alcoholic at certain times has no effective mental defense against the first drink. Except in a few rare cases, neither he nor any other human being can provide such a defense. His defense must come from a Higher Power.

CHAPTER THREE

We Agnostics

In the preceding chapters, you have learned something of alcoholism. We hope we have made clear the distinction between the alcoholic and the non-alcoholic.

If, when you honestly want to, you find you cannot quit entirely, or if, when drinking, you have little control over the amount you take, you are probably alcoholic. If that be the case, you may be suffering from an illness that only a spiritual experience will conquer.

To one who feels he is an atheist or agnostic such an experience seems impossible, but to continue as he is means disaster especially if he is an alcoholic of the hopeless variety. To be doomed to an alcoholic death or to live on a spiritual basis—not always easy alternatives to face.

But it isn't so difficult. About half our fellowship were of exactly that type. At first some of us tried to avoid the issue, hoping against hope we were not true alcoholics. But after a while we had to face the fact that we must find a spiritual basis of life—or else.

If a mere code of morals, or a better philosophy of life were sufficient to overcome alcoholism, many of us would have recovered long ago. But we found that such codes and philosophies did not save us, no matter how much we tried.

Our human resources, as marshaled by the will, were not sufficient; they failed utterly. Lack of power, that was our dilemma. We had to find a power by which we could live, and it had to be *A Power Greater Than Ourselves.* But where and how were we to find this Power?

Well, that's exactly what this book is about. Its main object is to enable you to find a Power greater than yourself, which will solve your problem. That means, of course, that we are going to talk about God. Here difficulty arises with agnostics. Many times we talk to a new man and watch his hope rise as we discuss his alcoholic problems and explain our fellowship. But his face falls when we speak of spiritual matters, especially when we mention God, for we have re-opened a subject that our man thought he had neatly evaded or entirely ignored.

We know how he feels. We have shared his honest doubt and prejudice. We looked upon this world of warring individuals, warring theological systems, and inexplicable calamity, with deep skepticism. We looked askance at many individuals who claimed to be godly. Yes, we of agnostic temperament have had these thoughts and experiences, and many more. Let us make haste to reassure you. We found that as soon as we were able to lay aside prejudice and express even a willingness to believe in a Power greater than ourselves, we commenced to get results, even though it was impossible for any of us to fully define or comprehend that Power, which is God.

Much to our relief, we discovered we did not need to consider another's conception of God. Our own conception, however inadequate, was sufficient to make the approach and to effect a contact with Him. As soon as we admitted the possible existence of a Creative Intelligence, a Spirit of the Universe underlying the totality of things, we began to be possessed of a new sense of power and direction, provided we took other simple steps. We found that God does not make too hard terms with those who seek Him. To us, the Realm of Spirit is broad, roomy, all inclusive; never exclusive or forbidding, to those who earnestly seek.

When, therefore, we speak to you of God, we mean your own conception of God. This applies, too, to other spiritual expressions that you find in this book. Do not let any prejudice you may have against spiritual terms deter you from honestly asking yourself what they mean to you. At the start, this is all we needed to commence spiritual growth, to effect our first conscious relation with God as we understood Him.

We needed to ask ourselves but one short question. "Do I now believe, or am I even willing to believe, that there is a Power greater than myself?" As soon as a man can say that he does believe, or is willing to believe, we emphatically assure him that he is on his way. It has been repeatedly proven among us that upon this simple cornerstone a wonderfully effective spiritual structure can be built.

Everybody nowadays believes in scores of assumptions for which there is good evidence, but no perfect visual proof. And does not science demonstrate that visual proof is the weakest proof? It is being constantly revealed, as mankind studies the material world, that outward appearances are not inward reality at all.

Instead of regarding ourselves as intelligent agents, spearheads of God's ever advancing Creation, we agnostics and atheists chose to believe that our human intelligence was the last word, the alpha and the omega, the beginning and end of all. Rather vain of us, wasn't it?

We who have traveled this dubious path beg you to lay aside prejudice, even against organized religion.

We have learned that whatever the human frailties of various faiths may be, those faiths have given purpose and direction to millions.

Our world has made more material progress in the last century than in all the millennia that went before. Almost everyone knows why. Students of ancient history tell us that the intellect of men in those days was equal to the best of today. Yet in ancient times material progress was painfully slow. The spirit of modern scientific inquiry, research, and invention was almost unknown. In the realm of the material, men's minds were fettered by superstition, tradition, and all sorts of fixed ideas. The contemporaries of Columbus thought a round earth preposterous. Others like them came near putting Galileo to death for his astronomical heresies. We asked ourselves this: are not some of us just as biased and unreasonable about the realm of the spirit as were the ancients about the realm of the material?

We had to ask ourselves why we shouldn't apply to our human problems this same readiness to change the point of view. We were having trouble with personal relationships, we couldn't control our emotional natures, we were prey to misery and depression, we couldn't make a living, we had a feeling of uselessness, we were full of fear, we were unhappy, we couldn't seem to be of real help to other people.

When we saw others solve their problems by simple reliance upon the Spirit of this universe, we had to stop doubting the power of God. Our ideas did not work. But the God idea did.

Logic is great stuff. We liked it. We still like it. It is not by chance we were given the power to reason, to examine the evidence of our senses, and to draw conclusions. That is one of man's magnificent attributes. We agnostically inclined would not feel satisfied with a proposal which does not lend itself to reasonable approach and interpretation. Hence we are at pains to tell why we think our present faith is reasonable, why we think it more sane and logical to believe than not to believe, why we say our former thinking was soft and mushy when we threw up our hands in doubt and said, "We don't know."

When we became alcoholics, crushed by a self-imposed crisis we could not postpone or evade, we had to fearlessly face the proposition that either God is everything or He is nothing. God either is, or He isn't. What was our choice to be?

Arrived at this point, we were squarely confronted with the question of faith. We couldn't duck the issue. Some of us had already walked far over the Bridge of Reason toward the desired shore of faith. The outlines and the promise of the New Land had brought lustre to tired eyes and fresh courage to flagging spirits. Friendly hands had stretched out in welcome. We were grateful that Reason had brought us so far. But somehow, we couldn't quite step ashore. Perhaps we had been leaning too heavily on Reason that last mile and we did not like to lose our support.

That was natural, but let us think a little more closely. Without knowing it, had we not been brought to where we stood by a certain kind of faith? For did we not believe in our own reasoning? Did we not have confidence in our ability to think? What was that but a sort of faith? Yes, we had been faithful, abjectly faithful to the God of Reason. So, in one way or another, we discovered that faith had been involved all the time!

Hence, we saw that reason isn't everything. Neither is reason, as most of us use it, entirely dependable, though it emanate from our best minds. We finally saw that faith in some kind of God was a part of our make-up, just as much as the feeling we have for a friend. Sometimes we had to search fearlessly, but He was there. He was as much a fact as we were. We found the Great Reality deep down within us. In the last analysis it is only there that He may be found. It was so with us.

We can only clear the ground a bit. If our testimony helps sweep away prejudice, enables you to think honestly, encourages you to search diligently within yourself, then if you wish you can join us on the Broad Highway. With this attitude you cannot fail. The consciousness of your belief is sure to come to you.

CHAPTER FOUR

How It Works

Rarely have we seen a person fail who has thoroughly followed our path. Those who do not recover are people who cannot or will not completely give themselves to this simple program, usually men and women who are constitutionally incapable of being honest with themselves. There are such unfortunates. They are not at fault; they seem to have been born that way. They are naturally incapable of grasping and developing a manner of living which demands rigorous honesty. There are those, too, who suffer from grave emotional and mental disorders, but many of them do recover if they have the capacity to be honest.

Remember that we deal with alcohol—cunning, baffling, powerful! Without help it is too much for us. But there is One who has all power—That One is God. May you find Him now!

Half measures availed us nothing. We stood at the turning point. We asked His protection and care with complete abandon.

Here are the steps we took, which are suggested as a Program of Recovery:

1. We admitted we were powerless over alcohol—that our lives had become unmanageable.
2. Came to believe that a Power greater than ourselves could restore us to sanity.
3. Made a decision to turn our will and our lives over to the care of God *as we understood Him.*
4. Made a searching and fearless moral inventory of ourselves.
5. Admitted to God, to ourselves, and to another human being the exact nature of our wrongs.
6. Were entirely ready to have God remove all these defects of character.
7. Humbly asked Him to remove our shortcomings.
8. Made a list of all persons we had harmed, and became willing to make amends to them all.
9. Made direct amends to such people wherever possible, except when to do so would injure them or others.
10. Continued to take personal inventory and when we were wrong promptly admitted it.

11. Sought through prayer and meditation to improve our conscious contact with God *as we understood Him* praying only for knowledge of His will for us and the power to carry that out.

12. Having had a spiritual experience as the result of these steps, we tried to carry this message to alcoholics, and to practice these principles in all our affairs.

Many of us exclaimed, "What an order! I can't go through with it." Do not be discouraged. No one among us has been able to maintain anything like perfect adherence to these principles. We are not saints. The point is, that we are willing to grow along spiritual lines. The principles we have set down are guides to progress. We claim spiritual progress rather than spiritual perfection.

Our description of the alcoholic, the chapter to the agnostic, and our personal adventures before and after make clear three pertinent ideas:

(a) That we were alcoholic and could not manage our own lives.

(b) That probably no human power could have relieved our alcoholism.

(c) That God could and would if sought.

Being convinced, *we were at step three*, which is that we decided to turn our will and our life over to God as we understood Him. Just what do we mean by that, and just what do we do?

The first requirement was that we be convinced that any life run on self-will could hardly be a success. On that basis we are almost always in collision with something or somebody, even though our motives are good. Most people try to live by self-propulsion. If his arrangements would only stay put, if only people would do as he wishes, the show would be great. Everybody, including himself, would be pleased.

What usually happens? The show doesn't come off very well. He begins to think life doesn't treat him right. He decides to exert himself some more. He becomes, on the next occasion, still more demanding or gracious, as the case may be. Still the play does not suit him. Admitting he may be somewhat at fault, he is sure that other people are more to blame. He becomes angry, indignant, self-pitying. What is his basic trouble? Is he not really a self-seeker even when trying to be kind? Is he not a victim of the delusion that he can wrest satisfaction and happiness out of this world if he only manages well?

Our troubles are basically of our own making. They arise out of ourselves, and the alcoholic is an extreme example of self-will run riot, though he usually doesn't think so. Above everything, we alcoholics must be rid of this selfishness. We must, or it kills us! God makes that possible. And there often seems no way of entirely getting rid of self without Him. Many of us had moral and philosophical convictions galore, but we could not live up to them even though we would have liked to. Neither could we reduce our self-centeredness much by wishing or trying on our own power. We had to have God's help.

This is the how and why of it. First of all, we had to quit playing God. It didn't work. Next, we decided that hereafter in this drama of life, God was going to be our Director. He is the Principal, we are His agent. He is the Father, and we are His children. Most good ideas are simple and this concept was the keystone of the new and triumphant arch through which we passed to freedom.

When we sincerely took such a position, all sorts of remarkable things followed. We had a new Employer. Being all powerful, He provided what we needed, if we kept close to Him and performed His work well. Established on such a footing we became less and less interested in ourselves, our little plans and designs. More and more we became interested in seeing what we could contribute to life. As we felt new power flow in, as we enjoyed peace of mind, as we discovered we could face life successfully, as we became conscious of His presence, we began to lose our fear of today, tomorrow, or the hereafter. We were reborn.

We were now at step three. Many of us said to our Maker, *as we understood Him:* "God, I offer myself to Thee—to build with me and to do with me as Thou wilt. Relieve me of the bondage of self, that I may better do Thy will. Take away my difficulties, that victory over them may bear witness to those I would help of Thy Power, Thy Love, and Thy Way of life. May I do Thy will always!" We thought well before taking this step making sure we were ready; that we could at last abandon ourselves utterly to Him.

The wording was, of course, quite optional so long as we expressed the idea, voicing it without reservation. This was only a beginning, though if honestly and humbly made, an effect, sometimes a very great one, was felt at once.

Next we launched on a course of vigorous action, the first step of which is a personal housecleaning, which many of us had never attempted. Though our decision was a vital and crucial step, it could have little permanent effect unless at once followed by a strenuous effort to face, and to be rid of, the things in ourselves that had been blocking us.

Therefore, we started upon a personal inventory. *This was step four.* A business that takes no regular inventory usually goes broke. Taking a commercial inventory is a fact-finding and a fact-facing process. It is an effort to discover the truth about the stock-in-trade. One object is to disclose damaged or unsalable goods, to get rid of them promptly, and without regret. If the owner of the business is to be successful, he cannot fool himself about values.

We did exactly the same thing with our lives. We took stock honestly. First, we searched out the flaws in our make-up which caused our failure. Being convinced that self, manifested in various ways, was what had defeated us, we considered its common manifestations.

Resentment is the "number one" offender. In dealing with resentments, we set them on paper. We listed people, institutions or principles with whom we were angry. We asked ourselves why we were angry. In most cases it was found that our self-esteem, our pocketbooks, our ambitions, our personal relationships (including sex) were hurt or threatened.

We went back through our lives. Nothing counted but thoroughness and honesty.

It is plain that a life that includes deep resentment leads only to futility and unhappiness. To the precise extent that we permit these, do we squander the hours that might have been worthwhile. But with the alcoholic whose hope is the maintenance and growth of a spiritual experience, this business of resentment is infinitely grave. It is fatal. For when harboring such feelings we shut ourselves off from the sunlight of the Spirit. The insanity of alcohol returns and we drink again. And with us, to drink is to die. If we were to live, we had to be free of anger. The grouch and the brainstorm were not for us. They may be the dubious luxury of normal men, but for alcoholics these things are poison.

We turned back to the list. We realized that the people who wronged us were perhaps spiritually sick. Though we did not like their symptoms and the way these disturbed us, they, like ourselves were sick, too. We asked God to help us show them the same tolerance, pity, and patience that we would cheerfully grant a sick friend. When a person offended we said to ourselves "This is a sick man. How can I be helpful to him? God save me from being angry. Thy will be done."

We avoid retaliation or argument. We wouldn't treat sick people that way. If we do, we destroy our chance of being helpful. We cannot be helpful to all people, but at least God will show us how to take a kindly and tolerant view of each and every one.

Referring to our list again, where had we been selfish, dishonest, self-seeking, and frightened? Though a situation had not been entirely our fault, we tried to disregard the other person involved entirely. Where were we to blame?

We reviewed our fears thoroughly. We put them on paper, even though we had no resentment in connection with them. We asked ourselves why we had them. Wasn't it because self-reliance failed us? Self-reliance was good as far as it went, but it didn't go far enough. Some of us once had great self-confidence, but it didn't fully solve the fear problem, or any other. When it made us cocky, it was worse.

Perhaps there is a better way—we think so. For we are now on a different basis; the basis of trusting and relying upon God. We trust infinite God rather than our finite selves. We are in the world to play the role He assigns. Just to the extent that we do as we think He would have us, and humbly rely on Him, does He enable us to match calamity with serenity.

We never apologize to anyone for depending upon our Creator. We can laugh at those who think spirituality the way of weakness. Paradoxically, it is the way of strength. The verdict of the ages is that faith means courage. All men of faith have courage. They trust their God. We never apologize for God. Instead we let Him demonstrate, through us, what He can do. We ask Him to remove our fear and direct our attention to what He would have us be. At once, we commence to outgrow fear.

Now about sex. Many of us needed an overhauling there. But above all, we tried to be sensible on this question. It's so easy to get way off the track. Here we find human opinions running to extremes—absurd extremes, perhaps. One set of voices cry that sex is a lust of our lower nature, a base necessity of procreation. Then we have the voices who cry for sex and more sex; who bewail the institution of marriage; who think that most of the troubles of the race are traceable to sex causes. They think we do not have enough of it, or that it isn't the right kind. They see its significance everywhere. One school would allow man no flavor for his fare and the other would have us all on a straight pepper diet. We want to stay out of this controversy. We do not want to be the arbiter of anyone's sex conduct. We all have sex problems. We'd hardly be human if we didn't. What can we do about them?

We reviewed our own conduct over the years past. Where had we been selfish, dishonest, or inconsiderate? Whom had we hurt? Did we unjustifiably arouse jealousy, suspicion or bitterness? Where were we at fault, what should we have done instead? We got this all down on paper and looked at it.

In this way we tried to shape a sane and sound ideal for our future sex life. Whatever our ideal turns out to be, we must be willing to grow toward it. We must be willing to make amends where we have done harm, provided that we do not bring about still more harm in so doing. In other words, we treat sex as we would any other problem. In meditation, we ask God what we should do about each specific matter. The right answer will come, if we want it.

To sum up about sex: we earnestly pray for the right ideal, for guidance in each questionable situation, for sanity, and for the strength to do the right thing. If sex is very troublesome, we throw ourselves the harder into helping others. We think of their needs and work for them. This takes us out of ourselves. It quiets the imperious urge, when to yield would mean heartache.

In this book you read again and again that faith did for us what we could not do for ourselves. We hope you are convinced now that God can remove whatever self-will has blocked you off from Him. If you have already made a decision, and an inventory of your grosser handicaps, you have made a good beginning. That being so, you have swallowed and digested some big chunks of truth about yourself.

CHAPTER FIVE

Into Action

Having made our personal inventory, what shall we do about it? We have been trying to get a new attitude, a new relationship with our Creator, and to discover the obstacles in our path. We have admitted certain defects; we have ascertained in a rough way what the trouble is; we have put our finger on the weak items in our personal inventory. Now these are about to be cast out. This requires action on our part, which, when completed, will mean that we have admitted to God, to ourselves, and to another human being, the exact nature of our defects. This brings us to *the fifth step* in the Program of Recovery: discussing our defects with another person.

We think we have done well enough in admitting these things to ourselves. There is doubt about that. In actual practice, we usually find a solitary self-appraisal insufficient. Many of us thought it necessary to go much further. We will be more reconciled to discussing ourselves with another person when we see good reasons to do so. The best reason first: if we skip this vital step, we may not overcome drinking. Time after time newcomers have tried to keep to themselves certain facts about their lives. Trying to avoid this humbling experience, they have turned to easier methods. Almost invariably they got drunk.

They took inventory all right, but hung on to some of the worst items in stock. They only *thought* they had lost their egoism and fear; they only *thought* they had humbled themselves. But they had not learned enough of humility, fearlessness, and honesty, in the sense we find necessary, until they told someone else *all* their life story.

More than most people, the alcoholic leads a double life. He is very much the actor. To the outer world he presents his stage character. This is the one he likes his fellows to see. He wants to enjoy a certain reputation, but knows in his heart he doesn't deserve it.

We must be entirely honest with somebody if we expect to live long or happily in this world. Rightly and naturally, we think well before we choose the person or persons with whom to take this intimate and confidential step. Those of us belonging to a religious denomination that requires confession, must, and of course, will want to go to the properly appointed authority whose duty it is to receive it. Though we have no religious connection, we may still do well to talk with someone ordained by an established religion. We often find such a person quick to see and understand our problem. Of course, we sometimes encounter people who do not understand alcoholics.

If we cannot, or would rather not do this, we search our acquaintance for a close-mouthed, understanding friend. Perhaps our doctor or psychologist will be the person. It may be one of our own family, but we cannot disclose anything to our spouses or our parents that will hurt them and make them unhappy. We have no right to save our own skin at another person's expense. Such parts of our story we tell to someone who will understand, yet be unaffected. The rule is we must be hard on ourself, but always considerate of others.

When we decide who is to hear our story, we waste no time. We have a written inventory, and we are prepared for a long talk. We pocket our pride and go to it, illuminating every twist of character, every dark cranny of the past. Once we have taken this step, withholding nothing, we are delighted. We can look the world in the eye. We can be alone at perfect peace and ease.

Returning home we find a place where we can be quiet for an hour, carefully reviewing what we have done. Carefully rereading the first five proposals we ask if we have omitted anything, for we are building an arch through which we shall walk a free man at last. Is our work solid so far? Are the stones properly in place? Have we skimped on the cement put into the foundation?

If we can answer to our satisfaction, we then look at *step six.* We have emphasized willingness as being indispensable. Are we now ready to let God remove from us all the things that we have admitted are objectionable?

When ready, we say something like this: "My Creator, I am now willing that you should have all of me, good and bad. I pray that you now remove from me every single defect of character that stands in the way of my usefulness to you and my fellows. Grant me strength, as I go out from here, to do your bidding. Amen." We have then completed *step seven.*

Now we need more action without which we find that "Faith without works is dead." Let's look at *steps eight and nine.* We have a list of all persons we have harmed, and to whom we are willing to make amends. We made it when we took inventory. We subjected ourselves to a drastic self-appraisal. Now we go out to our fellows and repair the damage done in the past. If we haven't the will to do this, we ask until it comes. Remember it was agreed at the beginning *we would go to any lengths for victory over alcohol.*

As we look over the list of business acquaintances and friends we have hurt, we may feel diffident about going to some of them on a spiritual basis. Let us be reassured. To some people we need not, and probably should not emphasize the spiritual feature on our first approach. We might prejudice them. At the moment we are trying to put our lives in order. But this is not an end in itself. Our real purpose is to fit ourselves to be of maximum service to God and the people about us. It is seldom wise to approach an individual, who still smarts from our injustice to him, and announce that we have gone religious. In the prize ring, this would be called leading with the chin. Why lay ourselves open to being branded fanatics or religious bores? We may kill a future opportunity to carry a beneficial message. But our man is sure to be impressed with a sincere desire to set right the wrong. He is going to be more interested in a demonstration of good will than in our talk of spiritual discoveries.

The spiritual life is not a theory. *We have to live it.* Unless one's family expresses a desire to live upon spiritual principles we think we ought not to urge them. We should not talk incessantly to them about spiritual matters. They will change in time. Our behavior will convince them more than our words. We must remember that ten or twenty years of drunkenness would make a skeptic out of anyone.

There may be some wrongs we can never fully right. We don't worry about them if we can honestly say to ourselves that we would right them if we could. Some people cannot be seen—we send them an honest letter. And there may be a valid reason for postponement in some cases. But we don't delay if it can be avoided. We should be sensible, tactful, and considerate and humble without being servile or scraping. As God's people we stand on our feet; we don't crawl before anyone.

This thought brings us to *step ten*, which suggests we continue to take personal inventory and continue to set right any new mistakes as we go along. We vigorously commenced this way of living as we cleaned up the past. We have entered the world of Spirit. Our next function is to grow in understanding and effectiveness. This is not an overnight matter. It should continue for our lifetime. Continue to watch for selfishness, dishonesty, resentment, and fear. When these crop up, we ask God at once to remove them. We discuss them with someone immediately and make amends quickly if we have harmed anyone. Then we resolutely turn our thoughts to someone we can help. Love and tolerance of others is our code.

Every day is a day when we must carry the vision of God's will into all of our activities. "How can I best serve Thee—Thy will (not mine) be done." These are thoughts that must go with us constantly. We can exercise our will power along this line all we wish. It is the proper use of the will.

Much has already been said about receiving strength, inspiration, and direction from Him who has all knowledge and power. If we have carefully followed directions, we have begun to sense the flow of His Spirit into us. To some extent we have become God-conscious. We have begun to develop this vital sixth sense. But we must go further and that means more action.

Step eleven suggests prayer and meditation. We shouldn't be shy on this matter of prayer. Better men than we are using it constantly. It works, if we have the proper attitude and work at it. It would be easy to be vague about this matter. Yet, we believe we can make some definite and valuable suggestions.

When we retire at night, we constructively review our day. Were we resentful, selfish, dishonest, or afraid? Do we owe an apology? Have we kept something to ourselves which should be discussed with another person at once? Were we kind and loving toward all? What could we have done better? Were we thinking of ourselves most of the time? Or were we thinking of what we could do for others, of what we could pack into the stream of life? But we must be careful not to drift into worry, remorse, or morbid reflection, for that would diminish our usefulness to others. After making our review we ask God's forgiveness and inquire what corrective measures should be taken.

On awakening let us think about the twenty-four hours ahead. We consider our plans for the day. Before we begin, we ask God to direct our thinking, especially asking that it be divorced from self-pity, dishonest or self-seeking motives. Under these conditions we can employ our mental faculties with assurance for after all God gave us brains to use. Our thought life will be placed on a much higher plane when our thinking is cleared of wrong motives.

We ask especially for freedom from self-will, and are careful to make no request for ourselves only. We may ask for ourselves, however, if others will be helped. We are careful never to pray for our own selfish ends. Many of us have wasted a lot of time doing that, and it doesn't work. You can easily see why.

We alcoholics are undisciplined. So we let God discipline us in the simple way we have just outlined.

But this is not all. There is action and more action. "Faith without works is dead." This brings us to the vital importance of step twelve: working with others.

Practical experience shows that nothing will so much ensure immunity from drinking as intensive work with other alcoholics. It works when other activities fail. This is our *twelfth suggestion:* Carry this message to other alcoholics! You can help when no one else can. You can secure their confidence when others fail. Remember they are very ill.

Life will take on new meaning. To watch people recover, to see them help others, to watch loneliness vanish, to see a fellowship grow up about you, to have a host of friends—this is an experience you must not miss. We know you will not want to miss it. Frequent contact with newcomers and with each other is the bright spot of our lives.

To be vital, faith must be accompanied by self-sacrifice and unselfish, constructive action. Let another see that you are not there to instruct him in religion. Admit that he probably knows more about it than you do, but call to his attention the fact that however deep his faith and knowledge, he could not have applied it, or he would not drink. Perhaps your story will help him see where he fails to practice the very precepts he knows so well. We represent no particular faith or denomination. We are dealing only with general principles common to most denominations.

Helping others is the foundation stone of your recovery. A kindly act once in a while isn't enough. You have to act the Good Samaritan every day, if need be. It may mean the loss of many nights' sleep, great interference with your pleasures, interruptions to your business. It may mean sharing your money and your home, counseling frantic wives and relatives, innumerable trips to police courts, sanitariums, hospitals, jails, and asylums. Your telephone may jangle at any time of the day or night.

Your job now is to be at the place where you may be of maximum helpfulness to others, so never hesitate to go anywhere, if you can be helpful. You should not hesitate to visit the most sordid spot on earth on such an errand. Keep on the firing line of life with these motives, and God will keep you unharmed.

We are careful never to show intolerance or hatred of drinking as an institution. Experience shows that such an attitude is not helpful to anyone. Every new alcoholic looks for this spirit among us and is immensely relieved when he finds we are not witch-burners. A spirit of intolerance might repel alcoholics whose lives could have been saved, had it not been for such stupidity. We would not even do the cause of temperate drinking any good, for not one drinker in a thousand likes to be told anything about alcohol by one who hates it.

Someday we hope that Alcoholics Anonymous will help the public to a better realization of the gravity of the alcoholic problem, but we shall be of little use if our attitude is one of bitterness or hostility. Drinkers will not stand for it.

After all, our problems were of our own making. Bottles were only a symbol. Besides, we have stopped fighting anybody or anything. We have to!

About the Authors

AA cofounder BILL WILSON (1895–1971), was the chief voice and writer behind *Alcoholics Anonymous*—often called "The Big Book"—on which he collaborated with many figures, including his wife and intellectual partner LOIS WILSON (1891–1988), his AA cofounder BOB SMITH (1879–1950), pioneering AA member HENRY PARKHURST (1895–1954), and a wide range of early AAs who contributed stories and strategies.

MITCH HOROWITZ, who abridged and introduced this volume, is the PEN Award-winning author of books including *Occult America* and *The Miracle Club: How Thoughts Become Reality*. *The Washington Post* says Mitch "treats esoteric ideas and movements with an even-handed intellectual studiousness that is too often lost in today's raised-voice discussions." Follow him @MitchHorowitz.

Printed in the USA
CPSIA information can be obtained
at www.ICGtesting.com
JSHW012045140824
68134JS00034B/3275

9 781722 500481